What is COPD?
Definition
Page 4

The clinical picture

Spectrum of COPD	Signs and symptoms	Risk factors
Pages 4-5	Page 5	Pages 5-6

Establishing the diagnosis

History / Spirometry	Classifying severity	When to refer	What else could it be?
Pages 6-11	Page 12	Page 13	Pages 14-15

Assessing the impact on the patient

Quality of life
Page 16

Breathlessness
Pages 17-18

Definition of COPD

- GOLD 2019: 'Chronic Obstructive Pulmonary Disease (COPD), a common preventable and treatable disease, is characterised by persistent respiratory symptoms and airflow limitation that is due to airway and/or alveolar abnormalities usually caused by significant exposure to noxious particles or gases.' (GOLD 2019 p4)

  - Airflow obstruction is defined as a reduced post-bronchodilator FEV_1/FVC ratio (where FVC is forced vital capacity), such that FEV_1/FVC is less than 0.7, (where FEV_1 is the forced expiratory volume in one second) and where FEV_1 is often less than 80% predicted
  - Airflow obstruction is due to a combination of airway and lung tissue damage
  - The damage is a result of chronic inflammation that differs from that seen in asthma
  - COPD is a common preventable and treatable disease with some significant extra-pulmonary effects that may contribute to severity in individual patients.

The clinical picture: spectrum of COPD

COPD is traditionally seen as an overlapping spectrum of disease processes.

Emphysema

Where emphysema predominates patients have relentlessly progressive breathlessness, unaccompanied by features of chronic bronchitis or asthma. Development of a barrel chest is a relatively early sign and is often easily seen because patients tend to be thin. Patients may naturally adopt pursed lip breathing to slow exhalation and prevent airway collapse.

Chronic bronchitis

Chronic bronchitis is defined by the production of sputum most days for three months of two consecutive years, where other causes of chronic sputum production have been excluded. The sputum of the smoker's cough indicates an abnormal pathological process. It is significant and may be an early warning sign of COPD. It may precede the development of airflow obstruction. Chronic bronchitis with airflow obstruction causes progressive, non-variable breathlessness.

NOTES
- See page 6 for differences between COPD and asthma
- Some individuals have asthma/COPD overlap (ACO). More information on ACO can be found in chapter 5 of this guideline: http://ginasthma.org/2017-gina-report-global-strategy-for-asthma-management-and-prevention/
- In the first instance COPD differs from asthma in that airflow obstruction can never be fully reversed

The Spectrum of COPD

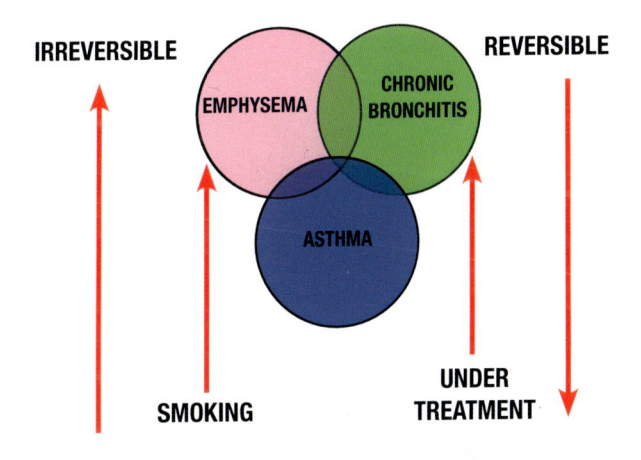

IRREVERSIBLE ↑

REVERSIBLE ↓

EMPHYSEMA — CHRONIC BRONCHITIS — ASTHMA

SMOKING ↑

UNDER TREATMENT ↑

Signs and symptoms suggesting COPD

COPD is a progressive disease passing through mild and moderate phases before becoming severe. Smokers often expect to have a cough and sputum production and do not consider these symptoms important. They frequently do not present until they have the significant breathlessness and extensive tissue damage associated with moderate to severe COPD. Unfortunately, this represents a missed opportunity for early diagnosis and intervention. Consider a diagnosis of COPD for people who are:

- over 35 and have risk factors for the disease with symptoms of
  - Breathlessness
  - Chronic cough
  - Regular sputum production
  - Frequent 'winter bronchitis'
  - Wheeze

The degree of airflow obstruction cannot be predicted from symptoms or signs.

Risk factors for developing COPD

- **The single most important cause of COPD is cigarette smoking**
- Any history of smoking should alert the health professional to the possibility of COPD
- In smokers at risk of developing COPD the greater the total tobacco exposure, the greater the risk
- Smoking history should include both the number of cigarettes smoked per day and for how long, as well as when stopped if applicable
- One pack year = 20 cigarettes smoked per day (1 pack) for one year
- Total pack years = $\dfrac{\text{no. of cigarettes smoked per day} \times \text{no. of years}}{20}$
- A tool that calculates this for you is available: www.smokingpackyears.com
- There are, of course, other forms of smoking tobacco that need to be considered. The following is a simple conversion that can be translated into pack years:

  1 pipe = 2.5 cigarettes
  1 cigar = 4 cigarettes
  1 cigarillo = 2 cigarettes

The COPD Pathway

Risk factors for developing COPD continued

- A smoking history of more than 15-20 pack years is considered significant but risk starts to increase after 10 pack years
- Other factors may also be important: history of repeated lower respiratory tract infection, poor nutrition, maternal smoking, lower socio-economic status, air pollution, and certain occupations, particularly those involving exposure to dusts and chemicals
- Alpha-1 antitrypsin deficiency is an inherited risk factor responsible for COPD in a small percentage of patients. Patients may develop severe COPD at a young age and with a light smoking history.

Establishing the diagnosis: history

- Patient's exposure to risk factors
- Past medical history including asthma, allergy, sinusitis, nasal polyps
- Childhood respiratory infections
- Family history of any respiratory disease
- Onset and pattern of symptoms
- History of respiratory infections
- Consider differential diagnosis (pages 14-15)

Establishing the diagnosis: spirometry

Objective assessment of lung function, measured by spirometry, is essential for accurate diagnosis of COPD. Primary care practitioners are in a key position to identify patients at risk of COPD. Early diagnosis and appropriate intervention can minimize the impact of the disease.

- The degree of airflow obstruction cannot be predicted from signs and symptoms
- Peak flow measurements are not useful in establishing a diagnosis of COPD. They do not distinguish between obstruction and restriction of airflow and they may seriously underestimate the degree of airflow obstruction in COPD
- Spirometry should be performed at the time of diagnosis and repeated at intervals to confirm the diagnosis and check disease progression
- Spirometry must be performed and interpreted by appropriately trained personnel certified and registered as competent.

Spirometry tracings

Spirometry measures the relaxed vital capacity (RVC, EVC or VC on different machines), the forced expiratory volume in one second (FEV_1) and the forced vital capacity (FVC).

Flow/Volume: The flow/volume trace plots expiratory flow rate (in litres/second) against the volume of air exhaled. The shape of the trace is helpful in identifying the type and severity of the ventilatory problem. The flow/volume trace on the right has a 'scooped out' shape. This indicates airflow obstruction.

NOTES
- Patients may assume that early symptoms of COPD are the 'expected' consequences of smoking and fail to mention them unless specifically asked
- Symptoms and clinical signs may suggest COPD but a firm diagnosis can only be made by objective measurement of airflow obstruction
- See page 12 for classifying the severity of COPD
- To distinguish between obstruction and restriction, see page 8

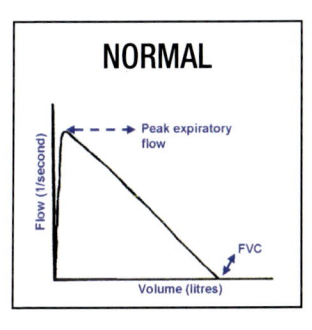

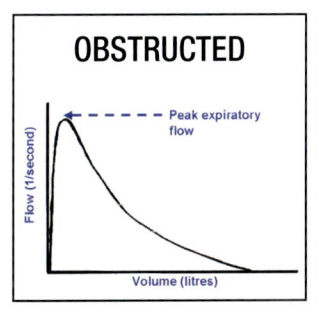

Volume/Time: Volume (in litres) is plotted on the vertical axis of the graph and time (in seconds) on the horizontal axis. The volume of FEV_1 and FVC can be measured and the FEV_1/FVC ratio calculated. In the normal trace, the patient forcibly exhaled three litres in one second (FEV_1) and a total of four litres (FVC). The FEV_1/FVC is therefore 75% (3 litres ÷ 4 litres x 100 = 75%).

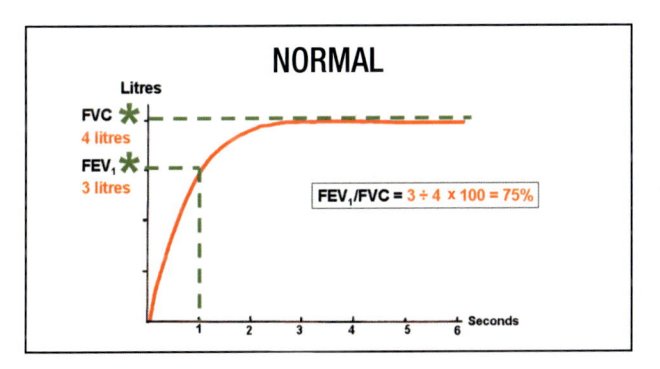

Recording spirometric measurements

Performing the test

- Measure height (no shoes) and record patient's age, gender and ethnicity
- Explain purpose and nature of test
- Explain and demonstrate technique
- Have patient sit comfortably throughout test in correct position.

NOTES
- Forced expiratory volume in the first second (FEV_1) is the measurement of choice in COPD as it is both reliable and reproducible
- Reductions in FEV_1 are directly related to prognosis – the worse the FEV_1 the worse the prognosis
- The severity of airflow obstruction is defined in terms of impairment of FEV_1 as a percentage of its predicted value – see classifying the severity of airflow obstruction on page 12
- For recording and assessing spirometric measurements ensure that equipment is regularly calibrated, cleaned and maintained and working correctly prior to use
- Incorrectly performed spirometry is meaningless; training in correct use is essential

7 The COPD Pathway

Using spirometry to confirm the diagnosis of COPD

If the clinical picture suggests COPD, post-bronchodilator spirometry should be carried out. In COPD, spirometric evidence of irreversible airflow obstruction will be seen. This means that there will be a reduced FEV_1/FVC ratio (less than 70% or 0.7) and the FEV_1 will normally (but not always) be below 80% of predicted. The FVC will often be normal. This pattern, in a quality assured trace, confirms the diagnosis of COPD in the presence of an appropriate history and symptoms.

Spirometry can also be used to diagnose other respiratory conditions, including asthma where reversibility will be seen. A systematic approach to carrying out and interpreting spirometry is important and the Quality Assured Diagnostic Spirometry document explains this in detail (see below).

For more information on spirometry see **https://www.pcc-cic.org.uk/sites/default/files/articles/attachments/spirometry_e-guide_1-5-13_0.pdf**

Defining the abnormality

- The pattern of values on spirometry indicates the type of impairment: obstructive disease (lungs may be normal size, but air cannot get out) vs restrictive disease (lungs may be smaller, but air can get out normally).

	Normal	**Obstructive Disease**	**Restrictive Disease**
FEV_1	Greater than 80% predicted	Usually less than 80% predicted	Less than 80% predicted
FVC	Greater than 80% predicted	Usually greater than 80% predicted but may be reduced in severe disease	Always less than 80% predicted
FEV_1/FVC	Greater than 0.7 (70%)	Less than 0.7 (70%)	Greater than 0.7 (70%)

Quality assured spirometry

Check patient demographics

Check patient demographics – the age, sex and height of an individual is what determines the predicted values for spirometry so the correct measurement of height and accurate entry of age, sex, height and ethnicity is fundamental.

Predicted values

The predicted values currently in use are from the European Community for Steel and Coal (ECSC) but have been superseded in newer spirometers by the Global Lung Function Initiative (GLI) values (**http://www.ers-education.org/guidelines/global-lung-function-initiative/resources-for-physicians.aspx**). The GLI values apply to people aged 3-95 years.

Technical acceptability

Inspect graphs to check they are free from faults and that the flow volume graph rises to a point (peak flow), comes downward smoothly and merges with the axis (FVC) with no abrupt end. The volume time should rise smoothly with a curve free from artefacts and continue for at least 6 seconds. There should be a minimum two-second plateau.

Number and quality of blows

There should be a minimum of three relaxed blows and three forced blows to a maximum of eight. Both the three relaxed and three forced blows should all be good quality i.e. no slow start, cough or abrupt end.

Reproducibility/repeatability

ARTP/BTS guidelines (http://www.artp.org.uk/en/professional/artp-standards/) require a maximum of 100mls or 5% between blows. This applies to VC, FVC and FEV_1. The GOLD guidelines allow for 150ml variation.

Interpretation of the ratio

Interpretation of the ratio involves checking the VC against the FVC and using the bigger value of the two. In some people with obstructive lung disease, air trapping results in a falsely reduced FVC. If the relaxed vital capacity is greater than the forced vital capacity this suggests that some air trapping has occurred and the FVC is not accurate and should not be used. In these cases, the best vital capacity from a relaxed blow should be used.

Normally, a reduced ratio (<70% or 0.7) suggests obstruction. In the elderly, however, using a fixed ratio of 0.7 (70%) may misdiagnose respiratory conditions in lungs that have lost elasticity due to the normal ageing process and consideration should be given to using the lower limits of normal (LLN) values. However, GOLD (2019) does not support use of the LLN and continues to advocate the fixed ratio of 70%. This remains a contentious issue in the respiratory world.

Severity of obstruction

Severity of obstruction – is defined by using the FEV_1. If irreversible obstruction is present and the symptoms and history support a diagnosis of COPD it is important to remember that the severity of COPD is not defined by the degree of airflow limitation but by symptoms and exacerbation history (GOLD 2019).

NOTES
- Abnormal spirometry usually precedes the development of symptoms. See Signs and Symptoms, page 5; Spirometry, pages 6-11
- Normal (predicted) lung volumes for FEV_1 and FVC are based on large adult population studies. Values of 20% on either side of predicted are considered normal. There are no population studies of subjects over 70 years of age so predicted values are based on estimates of how lungs age
- Normal values for height, age, gender and ethnicity are programmed into most electronic spirometers

Reversibility

Reversibility is measured as an improvement in FEV_1 comparing pre and post-bronchodilator readings. BTS/SIGN guidelines (https://www.brit-thoracic.org.uk/document-library/clinical-information/asthma/btssign-asthma-guideline-2016/) state that reversibility is present if there is a 12% change plus 200mls or more increase in FEV_1.

Reversibility testing

The guidelines do not recommend reversibility testing as a routine diagnostic procedure in COPD.

The role of reversibility testing is to help differentiate between asthma and COPD in cases where the clinical history is not clear.

Bronchodilator reversibility

Spirometry should be measured before and after an adequate dose of inhaled bronchodilator, e.g.

- Salbutamol, four puffs via MDI and spacer

Measure lung function
- 15 minutes after inhalation of $beta_2$ agonist

- A short-acting muscarinic antagonist could also be used, in which case the lung function should be measured 30-45 minutes post bronchodilator.

NOTES
- Consider CXR in any patient presenting atypically or with additional symptoms

KEY RECOMMENDATION
Streamlined referral pathways should be developed for tests not available or appropriate in Primary Care.

NICE diagnosis algorithm

Suspected COPD

- >35 years
- Smoker/ex-smoker
- Exertional breathlessness / chronic cough / regular sputum production / frequent winter 'bronchitis' / wheeze
- No clinical features of asthma

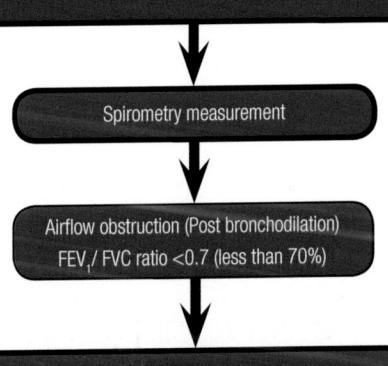

↓

Spirometry measurement

↓

Airflow obstruction (Post bronchodilation) FEV_1/ FVC ratio <0.7 (less than 70%)

↓

Diagnostic doubt? Consider:

- Clinically significant COPD unlikely if FEV_1 and FEV_1/FVC return to normal with treatment. Suspect asthma and follow BTS/SIGN asthma guidelines.

Asthma may be present if:

- FEV_1 improves by 200ml or more in response to bronchodilators
- Serial PEF shows diurnal or day-to-day variability
- FEV_1 improves by 200ml or more following 30mg prednisolone for 2 weeks or an inhaled corticosteroid taken for 6 weeks

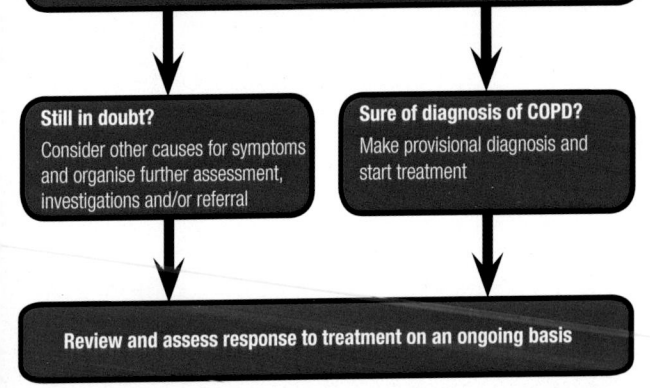

↓ ↓

Still in doubt?
Consider other causes for symptoms and organise further assessment, investigations and/or referral

Sure of diagnosis of COPD?
Make provisional diagnosis and start treatment

↓

Review and assess response to treatment on an ongoing basis

Classification of severity of airflow obstruction

The degree of airflow obstruction may help clinicians to predict exacerbation and mortality risk.

However, COPD is a multicomponent disorder and classification of severity of COPD on FEV_1 alone will not adequately assess the impact of the disease in an individual patient.

NICE(2010)/GOLD(2019)
Stage 1 >80%
Stage 2 >50-79%
Stage 3 >30-49%
Stage 4 <30%

Assessment of severity of COPD

There is poor correlation between lung function and disability.

Some patients with mild lung function impairment can be significantly disabled whereas some people with severe lung function impairment continue to work and function normally.

- COPD is a multicomponent disorder and classification of severity on FEV_1 alone will not adequately assess the impact of the disease in an individual patient

- Assessment of severity should include the degree of airflow obstruction and disability the frequency of exacerbations and other known factors affecting the prognosis,
  - FEV_1
  - T_LCO Gas transfer
  - Breathlessness
    – MRC (mMRC) scale (page 17)
  - Health status (page 16)
  - Exercise capacity
  - Body Mass Index
  - Blood gases–partial pressure of arterial oxygen (P_aO_2)
  - Cor pulmonale

Refer to a respiratory specialist in the following circumstances:

- Diagnostic uncertainty, or if the patient requests a second opinion
- Severe COPD 'not responding to treatment'
- FEV_1 declining rapidly
- Onset of cor pulmonale, presence of cyanosis and ankle oedema or pulse oximetry less than 92% when clinically stable
- Assessment for oxygen therapy, long-term nebuliser therapy or long-term oral corticosteroid therapy
- Assessment for surgery for bullous lung disease, lung volume reduction surgery or lung transplantation
- Symptoms disproportionate to lung function deficit/dysfunctional breathing
- Haemoptysis present
- Patient under 40 years or a family history of alpha-1 antitrypsin deficiency
- Frequent infective episodes. This could indicate bronchiectasis.

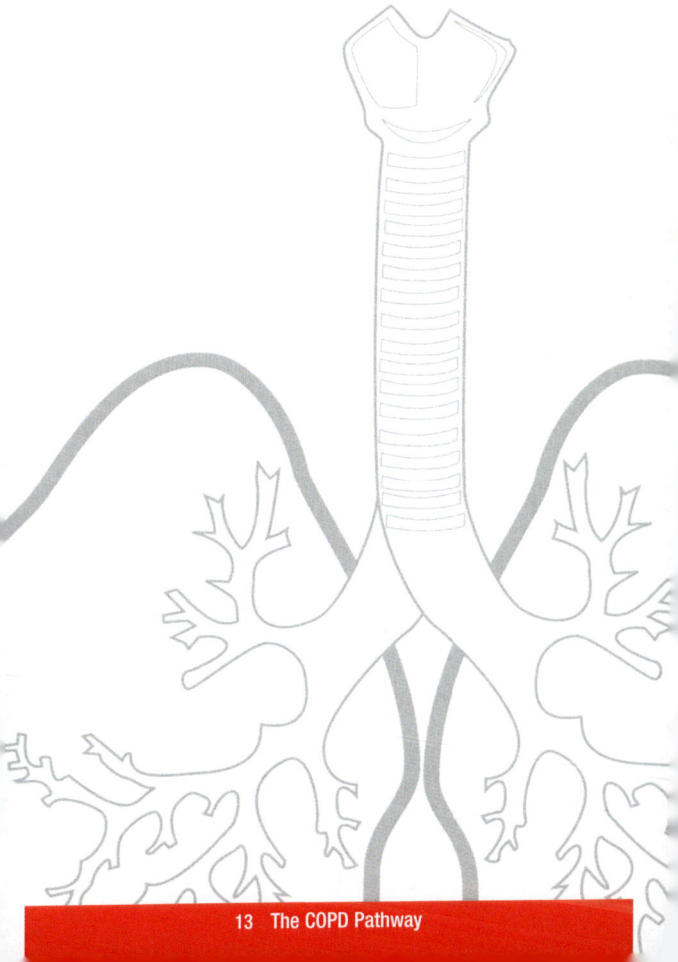

What else could it be?

COPD may be difficult to differentiate from other diseases, e.g. asthma, ischaemic heart disease or lung cancer – or may coexist with them.

When there is any doubt about the diagnosis, the patient must be referred for a specialist opinion.

Asthma

	COPD	ASTHMA
Smoker or ex-smoker	Nearly all	Possibly
Symptoms under the age of 35 years	Rarely	Often
Chronic, productive cough	Common	Uncommon except during exacerbations
Breathlessness	Common presenting symptom	Variable
Nocturnal waking with breathlessness and wheeze	Less common	Common
Day-to-day or diurnal variability of symptoms	Uncommon	Common
Family history of atopy or asthma	Uncommon	Common
Response to treatment	Partial	Good – in the majority of cases

Lung cancer

- Like COPD, associated with history of smoking
- Smokers with COPD are at greater risk of lung cancer than smokers without COPD
- Usually (but not always) visible on chest X-ray
- Never ascribe haemoptysis to COPD without excluding lung cancer
- Weight loss, finger clubbing and enlarged supraclavicular nodes are other clinical signs of lung cancer.

Cardiac disease

- Often co-exists with COPD, with similar symptoms, so ask specifically about previous history of angina, myocardial infarction and hypertension
- Chest X-ray, BNP (b-type natriuretic peptide) blood test, echocardiography and ECG may help differentiate between COPD and left-sided heart failure
- Use of cardiac drugs (e.g. diuretics, beta blockers, ACE inhibitors, nitrates, digoxin) may indicate previous history of angina, myocardial infarction or hypertension
- Ankle swelling may indicate cor pulmonale or congestive heart failure.

Other lung problems

- Tuberculosis, pulmonary fibrosis
- Excessive purulent sputum production (more than half a cup/day) may indicate bronchiectasis.

Anaemia

- Haemoglobin level will be reduced if breathlessness is due to anaemia
- Polycythaemia (abnormally raised haemoglobin levels) may be present in in people with COPD who are chronically hypoxic.

Investigations

At the time of diagnosis, in addition to spirometry some patients should have
- A chest X-ray – to help exclude other pathologies
- Full blood count – to identify anaemia or polycythaemia
- ECG to help exclude cardiac arrhythmias or other cardiac causes.

Additional investigations (or referral for further investigation) may need to be considered in some patients:
- Serial peak expiratory flow measurement – to exclude asthma
- Pulse oximetry – cyanosis, or FEV_1 less than 50% predicted, or features of cor pulmonale
- Blood test for alpha-1 antitrypsin – if early onset, light smoking history or family history
- Gas transfer (TLCO) – to aid diagnosis of COPD
- CT scanning – chest X-ray abnormalities, possible bronchiectasis
- ECG and/or echocardiogram – features of cardiac disease or cor pulmonale
- Sputum culture – persistent purulent sputum

Assessing the impact on the patient

- Some patients with mild lung function impairment can be significantly disabled
- Patients are not concerned with the level of their FEV_1, but with how far they can walk and with their ability to perform everyday tasks
- Disability is defined as an inability to perform activities of daily living
- The impact of COPD on psychological, sexual and social functioning (health status/quality of life) should be assessed regularly as these may be improved by appropriate management
- It is important to assess the impact of COPD on the patient from the beginning so that the effects of interventions can be evaluated and disease progression monitored.

Measuring health status

The COPD assessment test (CAT) is a validated tool which can be used to assess health status in people with COPD. It is a shorter, modified version of St George's Respiratory Questionnaire and is suitable for use in primary care.

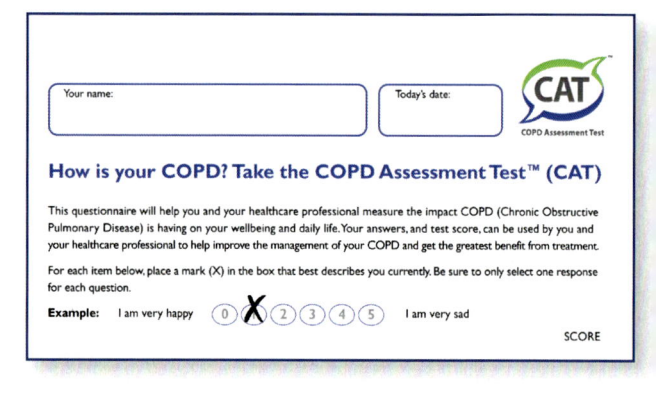

CAT
COPD Assessment Test

Your name: Today's date:

How is your COPD? Take the COPD Assessment Test™ (CAT)

This questionnaire will help you and your healthcare professional measure the impact COPD (Chronic Obstructive Pulmonary Disease) is having on your wellbeing and daily life. Your answers, and test score, can be used by you and your healthcare professional to help improve the management of your COPD and get the greatest benefit from treatment.

For each item below, place a mark (X) in the box that best describes you currently. Be sure to only select one response for each question.

Example: I am very happy (0) (X) (2) (3) (4) (5) I am very sad

SCORE

To view the COPD Assessment Test (CAT) visit www.catestonline.org

Quality of life – possible questions to ask:

- What are the two daily activities that cause the most breathlessness or distress?
- What is your overall level of fatigue?
- Are you upset or frightened by your episodes of breathlessness?
- Do you feel in control of your breathlessness or fatigue?
- Do you feel a burden to family, friends, and neighbours?
- Do you feel that it is safe for you to exercise?

Depression and anxiety are common in patients with severe COPD and impact significantly on health status. Treatment with conventional antidepressants and anxiolytics is safe and effective.

Measuring breathlessness – MRC dyspnoea scale

It is important to assess breathlessness regularly.
These scales can be used in both primary and secondary care settings.
N.B. The mMRC (GOLD 2019) is the European version of the MRC dyspnoea scale which scores 0-4 rather than the UK's 1-5).

1	Not troubled by breathlessness except on strenuous exercise
2	Short of breath when hurrying or walking up a slight hill
3	Walks slower than contemporaries on level ground because of breathlessness, or has to stop for breath when walking at own pace
4	Stops for breath after walking about 100 metres or after a few minutes on level ground
5	Too breathless to leave the house, or breathless when dressing or undressing

Oxygen cost diagram

- Patient marks a point on the line opposite where s/he becomes breathless
- Ability score is distance in cm from zero point

10

brisk walk uphill
medium walk uphill

brisk walk on the level

Borg scale

Patient scores their breathlessness during a particular activity

0. Nothing at all
   Very, very slight (just noticeable)
1. Very slight
2. Slight
3. Moderate
4. Somewhat severe
5. Severe (heavy)
6.
7. Very severe
8.
9. Very, very severe (almost maximal)
10. Maximal

slow walk uphill — heavy shopping
medium walk

light shopping

bed making
washing yourself

slow walking on the level
sitting

sleeping

0

Measuring walking distance

These tests form part of the assessment for pulmonary rehabilitation and can be used to measure response to therapy (e.g. inhaler therapy or ambulatory oxygen).

NOTES
- Formal questionnaires are available for health status evaluation, e.g. St. George's Respiratory Questionnaire; Breathing Problems Questionnaire, and form part of assessment and evaluation of pulmonary rehabilitation
- Longer questionnaires, such as the St. George's Respiratory Questionnaire, are often used for research studies, whereas shorter ones such as the CAT can be used effectively in primary care

Assessing the impact on the patient continued

Six-minute walking test:

- Have patient walk as far as possible, indoors on the flat, in six minutes
- Allow patient to stop as needed. Encourage patient to make best effort
- Record distance on second attempt (after a practice)
- Have patient assess degree of breathlessness before and after walk using a 10cm visual-analogue scale:

| Extremely short of breath | 0 ——————————— 10 | No shortness of breath |

- Evaluate what limits exercise i.e. breathlessness, leg fatigue, dizziness.

Shuttle walk test:

- Patient walks between two cones placed 10 metres apart (a shuttle) at a pace set by 'bleeps' on a tape recording
- Pace of walk is increased at a set rate
- Patient continues until s/he is unable to keep up or is forced to stop because of breathlessness or tiredness
- Record the number of completed shuttles.

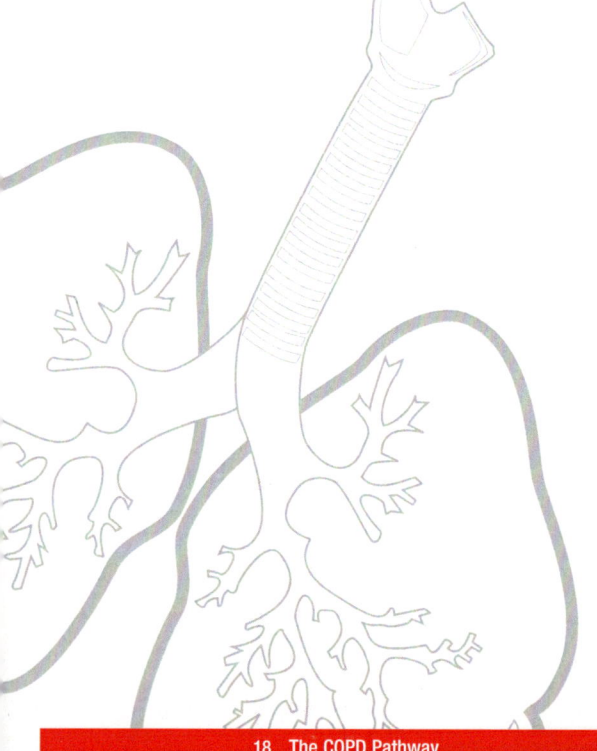

Promoting good self-management

- Patients with COPD often have low self-esteem, feeling that the disease is self-inflicted and that nothing can be done to help them
- The aim is to focus on the positive changes that can be made by the health care team in active partnership with the patient
- Good self-management can reduce complications, promote symptom control and improve quality of life
- It is never too late to stop smoking
- Patients should be encouraged to remain active and to maintain social contacts.

Explaining the causes of COPD
Page 20

Smoking and the decline of lung function
Page 21

Stopping smoking
Pages 22-25

Improving exercise tolerance

Pulmonary rehabilitation	Exercise reconditioning	Breathing exercises
Pages 26-27	Pages 28-29	Pages 30-32

Explaining the causes of COPD

Changes in the lungs

- It is important to help patients understand the changes that have taken place in their lungs
- In chronic bronchitis, the small airways become narrower and distorted, reducing the flow of air. Excess mucus production reduces airflow further
- In emphysema there is damage to the air sacs in the lungs so that there is reduced ability to absorb oxygen. In addition there is a loss of elastic recoil in the tissues supporting the airways, which leads to airway collapse and air trapping on exhalation
- These changes mean that it becomes harder to breathe out, the lungs become over – inflated and the size of each breath in is reduced
- Considerable structural changes can take place in the lungs without the individual noticing
- These structural changes are all irreversible, but at any point it is possible to minimize further damage.

What causes the lung changes?

- It is very important that patients understand that SMOKING is almost invariably the cause of COPD; it is much more important than any other risk factors
- Unless patients understand and accept the fundamental role of smoking in causing their disease, they are unlikely to stop smoking
- Listen to and acknowledge the patient's anxieties while stressing that although COPD cannot be cured, the symptoms can be managed and improved.

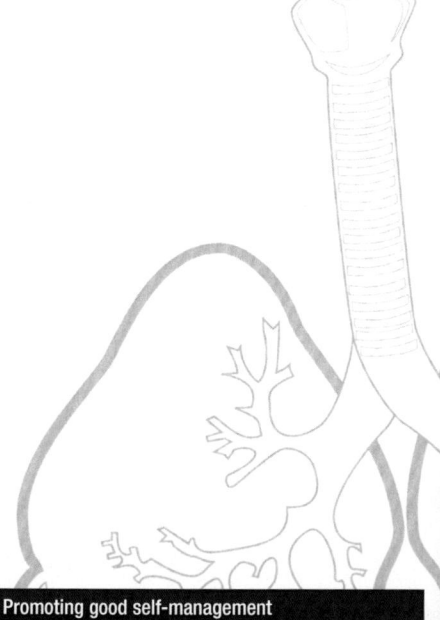

Smoking and the decline of lung function

Influence of smoking on FEV_1

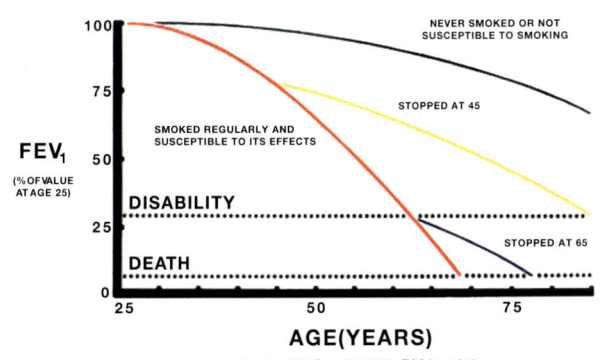

FEV_1 (% OF VALUE AT AGE 25)

- NEVER SMOKED OR NOT SUSCEPTIBLE TO SMOKING
- STOPPED AT 45
- SMOKED REGULARLY AND SUSCEPTIBLE TO ITS EFFECTS
- DISABILITY
- STOPPED AT 65
- DEATH

AGE (YEARS)

Fletcher CM, Peto R (1977), *BMJ* 1: 1645

- FEV_1 normally declines after age 25 at a rate of 25-30ml per year
- Smoking in susceptible individuals greatly accelerates this age-related change, to as much as 60ml per year
- Although the structural changes in COPD produced by cigarette smoking are irreversible, stopping smoking slows the decline to the normal rate
- Even when the smoker is disabled by COPD, smoking cessation can improve life expectancy and quality of life
- The key message for patients is:

IT IS NEVER TOO LATE TO STOP SMOKING!

NOTES
- For stopping smoking, see pages 22-25

21 Promoting good self-management

Stopping smoking

The single most important health intervention that health professionals can make is to help patients stop smoking.

Educate about the impact of smoking

Smoking is the primary cause of preventable illness and premature death, accounting for approximately 100,000 deaths a year in the United Kingdom. For every death caused by smoking, approximately 20 smokers are suffering from a smoking-related disease.
(ASH 2017 http://ash.org.uk)

- Compared to non-smokers, smokers are at greater risk of peptic ulcer disease, COPD and many cancers
- Cardiovascular risk is increased
- Erectile dysfunction is more common in smokers
- Over 7000 irritants and toxins have been identified in cigarette smoke including acetone, carbon monoxide, benzene and N-nitrosamine carcinogens
- Cigarettes deliver a bolus of nicotine straight to the brain with each inhalation. Nicotine delivery to the brain is quicker than if it were injected intravenously. It is this rapid and intense delivery of nicotine that feeds the addictive process.

Targeting the right patients: readiness to quit

Stopping smoking involves making a profound lifestyle change.
There are stages in the cycle of change and relapse is a normal part of the process.

Cycle of Change

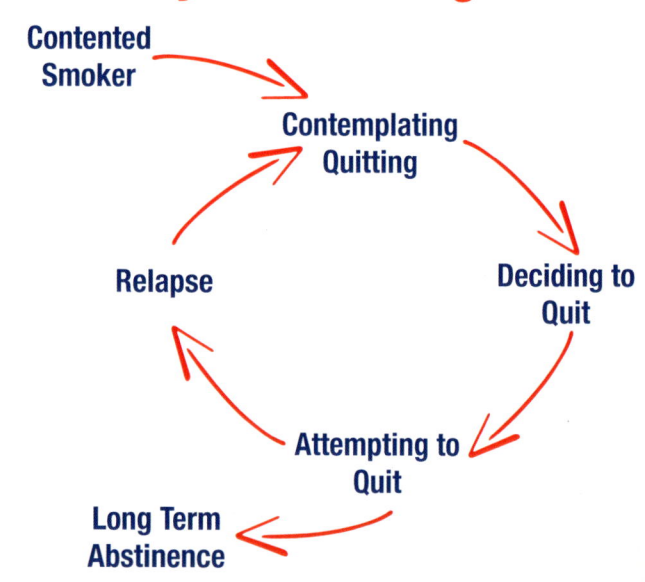

- Contented Smoker
- Contemplating Quitting
- Deciding to Quit
- Attempting to Quit
- Long Term Abstinence
- Relapse

Adapted from Prochaska 1986
Thorax 53 (Suppl 5), S1-S18

Brief intervention

Even the contented smoker who is unwilling to quit should be offered at least a brief intervention

- Provide information relevant to patient's situation
- Identify short-and long-term risks for patient and for others
- Help patient identify benefits of quitting
- Clarify barriers to quitting and ways they might be overcome
- Identify and address ambivalence.

The 5As Approach

- **Ask:** Identify all tobacco users in house
- **Advise** the patient to quit using clear, strong and personalised messages
- **Assess** patient's willingness to make a quit attempt in next 30 days
- **Assist** in developing a quit plan (see below)
- **Arrange** follow-up contact.

Elements of the quit plan

Prepare to quit

- Set the quit date (within two weeks is ideal)
- Tell family and friends; elicit support
- Anticipate challenges; remove tobacco.

Provide practical counselling

- Total abstinence may be best for most people, others may prefer to reduce gradually
- Review past quit attempts for critical success factors
- Anticipate triggers and challenges such as alcohol, other smokers (particularly within the home).

Mobilise support

- Support within the workplace and in the community is critical.

Recommend pharmacotherapy (see next page)

Provide supplementary materials

- Resources are available online and in print.

Preventing relapse

- Regular praise and encouragement
- Follow-up visits or phone calls
- Personalised problem solving i.e. depression, weight gain, withdrawal symptoms
- Warn patients that their cough may actually increase for a while immediately after quitting.

Pharmacotherapy for smoking cessation

- All smokers should be offered pharmacotherapy to assist with quitting
- Contraindications and cost vs benefit need to be considered in those smoking fewer than ten cigarettes/day, in pregnant or breastfeeding women and in adolescent smokers.

Nicotine replacement therapy (NRT)

NRT aims to partially replace nicotine from cigarettes. It provides a background level of nicotine at a lower dose and reduces craving and withdrawal symptoms. It is less suitable for genuinely light smokers and is not a panacea. It will not work if the smoker is not committed to stopping.

Nicotine is delivered at a slower rate from NRT products and does not 'feed' the nicotine addiction in the same way as cigarettes.

NRT can also be used as part of a 'cut down, then stop' strategy.

- Nicotine transdermal patches
  5mg, 10mg, 15mg – 16 hour patches 7mg, 14mg, 21mg
- Nicotine chewing gum – 2mg, 4mg
- Nicotine sub-lingual tablets – 2mg tablets
- Nicotine lozenges – 1mg, 1.5mg, 2mg, 4mg lozenges
- Nicotine inhalator – 10mg, 15mg inhalation cartridges
- Nicotine nasal spray – 0.5mg per puff metered nasal spray
- Mouth spray 1mg
- Orodispersible strips 2.5mg

Bupropion (Zyban)

Bupropion is only available on prescription and is licensed for smokers over the age of 18 as an aid to smoking cessation. It is thought to work by inhibiting some of the chemical messengers in the brain that are involved in addiction and withdrawal.
There are some important contraindications and cautions:

- Current seizure disorder (e.g. epilepsy)
- History of seizures
- Concurrent use of drugs that lower the seizure threshold
  (e.g. theophylline, monoamine oxidase inhibitors)
- Alcohol abuse or acute alcohol withdrawal
- Extreme caution should be exercised in patients who have a history of bipolar disorder, severe head injury, anorexia.

Full knowledge of the patient's medical and drug history is essential and the data sheet should be consulted for a full list of cautions and contraindications.

Varenicline

Varenicline (UK trade name Champix) is licensed for smokers over the age of 18 as an aid to smoking cessation. It is recommended for use alongside regular behavioural support for smoking cessation.

- Varenicline binds directly on the nicotine receptors, partially mimicking the effects of nicotine. This effectively reduces the cravings experienced by people when they quit and they will often describe being disinterested in cigarettes soon after starting on treatment
- By blocking the nicotine receptors in the brain, varenicline reduces the ability of nicotine from cigarettes to have an effect. This means that if people smoke while on treatment, they will not get any pleasure from their cigarette. This is a 'back up' effect to that of reducing the desire to smoke
- Varenicline is a prescription-only medicine which is available in two–and four–week packs; the usual course of treatment lasts for 12 weeks
- After 12 weeks if the quit attempt has been successful, treatment should be withdrawn. Tapering of the dose following a successful quit attempt is unnecessary; by 12 weeks the nicotine receptors in the brain have been 'deactivated' and will no longer crave nicotine
- Occasionally a further 12 weeks of treatment can be prescribed as this has been shown to improve quit rates in highly dependent smokers
- The most common side effects of varenicline are nausea, headaches and sleep disturbance. For most people these effects are tolerable and/or transient.

It is extremely important to note that most people who start on varenicline fail to complete the course of treatment. This may be because they become over-confident once the drug starts to work and they find that they have no interest in smoking. It is vital, therefore, to inform smokers that the 12-week course of treatment should be completed, no matter how confident they are feeling, in order to maximise the chances of long-term success.

https://www.nice.org.uk/guidance/qs43

NICE (2013) tobacco harm reduction: htts://www.nice.org.uk/ph45

NICE (2018) Overview Stop smoking interventions and services
https://www.nice.org.uk/guidance/ng92

Improving exercise tolerance

Effect of COPD on activity

Fear and distress induced by breathlessness often results in COPD patients avoiding activity. This leads to weakness of non-respiratory muscles and loss of cardiovascular fitness, causing worsening breathlessness.

Pulmonary rehabilitation

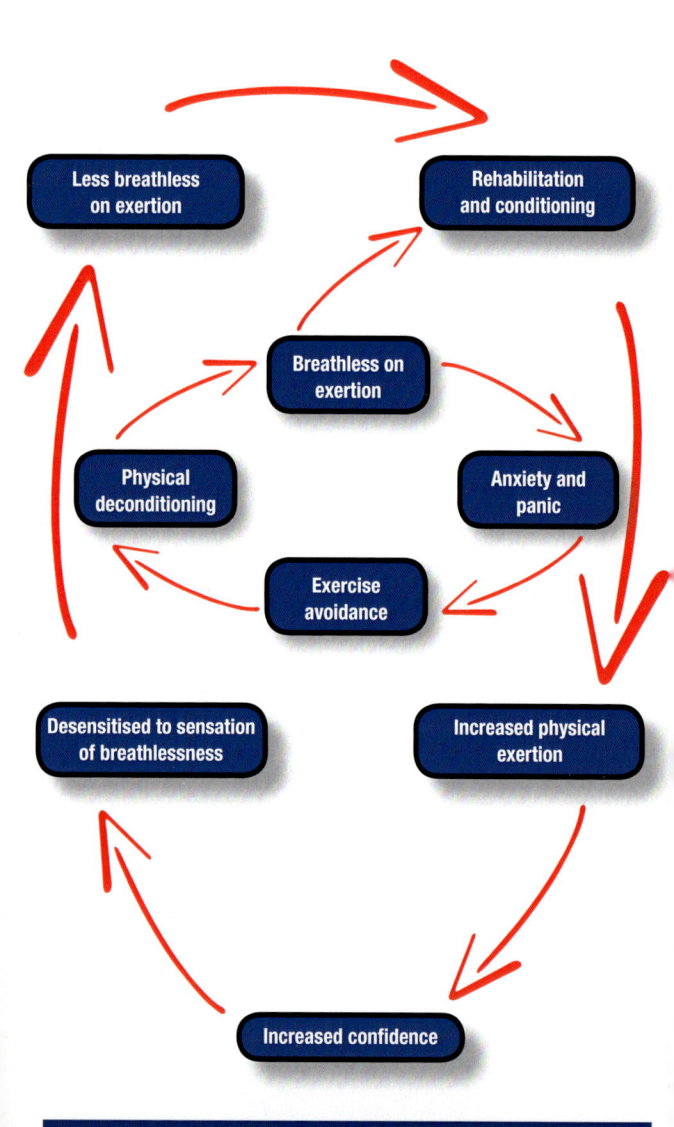

- Less breathless on exertion
- Rehabilitation and conditioning
- Breathless on exertion
- Anxiety and panic
- Exercise avoidance
- Physical deconditioning
- Increased physical exertion
- Desensitised to sensation of breathlessness
- Increased confidence

Exercise and rehabilitation continued

- Pulmonary rehabilitation is an organised and structured programme of exercise and education, delivered by a multi-disciplinary team. It aims to maximise a patient's physical and social functioning and improve their self-management skills
- The aim is to retrain deconditioned muscles, improve overall fitness and improve efficiency of oxygen use
- The core of a programme is individually prescribed exercise. Most programmes also include medical management, education, emotional support, breathing retraining and nutritional counselling
- Regular exercise, under supervision, reinforces the message that breathlessness is not harmful
- Regular exercise, to the point of breathlessness, may blunt the sensation of breathlessness enabling the patient to do more.

Documented outcomes of such programmes include
- Improved exercise tolerance
- Improved functional capacity
- Decreased use of health service resources
- Improved quality of life

- The GOLD 2019 and NICE 2018 guidelines recommend that pulmonary rehabilitation should be
  - Available to all suitable patients
  - Offered to all COPD patients who consider themselves functionally disabled
  - Available in a range of settings (including, potentially, the home [GOLD 2019, p57])

Patient selection

- All patients benefit from exercise programmes. They improve exercise tolerance and reduce symptoms of dyspnoea and fatigue
- The severity of COPD is not a factor in patient selection, though the nature of the exercise programme will need to be tailored to the patient's abilities
- Local services may be restricted to people with an MRC score of 3 (mMRC 2) or worse.

Advising patients about exercise

- Advise all COPD patients to maintain, and preferably increase their activity levels
- Advise patients that breathlessness is not harmful and it is safe and beneficial to get a little breathless
- Refer to a pulmonary rehabilitation programme if patients feel they are functionally disabled by COPD or grade themselves as MRC grade 3 or above (see page 17) Refer to a pulmonary rehabilitation programme within four weeks of a hospital discharge following an acute exacerbation
- If this is not possible, advise on simple exercises that can be built up slowly over three to four weeks and continued at home. (See pages 28-29.)
- 'Exercise on prescription' programmes are helpful for patients with mild/moderate COPD
- Self-help groups such as the British Lung Foundation's 'Breathe Easy' groups which meet regularly may provide mutual encouragement and support.

NOTES
- The British Lung Foundation runs Breathe Easy groups to support people with lung conditions such as COPD www.lunguk.org

Exercises for people with COPD

Refer patients with moderate/severe COPD who are MRC grade 3 or above (page 17) for pulmonary rehabilitation. If this is not available, the following cycle of gentle exercises, carried out daily, may be beneficial.

1. Shoulder shrugging:

Circle shoulder girdle forward, down, backwards and up. Keep timing constant, allowing two full seconds per circle and relax throughout. Continue for 30 seconds. Repeat the exercise three times with short rest intervals between sets.

2. Full arm circling:

One arm at a time, pass arm as near as possible to the side of the head, circle arm in as large a circle as possible (ten seconds/circle). Repeat for forty seconds. Repeat exercise three times with short rest intervals between repetitions. Repeat with other arm.

3. Increasing arm circles:

Hold arm away from body at shoulder height. Progressively increase size of circles for a count of six circles in ten seconds; then decrease for a further count of six. Repeat for 40 seconds. Repeat with other arm.

4. Abdominal exercise:

Sitting in a chair, tighten abdominal muscles, hold for a count of four; then release over four seconds to starting position. Repeat continuously for 30 seconds. Perform the procedure three times with a short rest period after each procedure.

5. Wall press–ups:

Stand with feet a full arm's length distance from the wall; place hands on wall and bend at elbow until nose touches the wall; push arms straight again allowing eight seconds from start to completion. Repeat for 40 seconds continuously to a total of five repetitions. Repeat three times with a short rest period after each procedure.

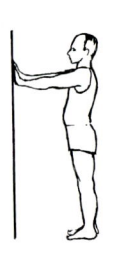

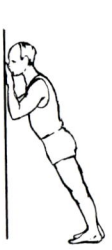

Exercises for people with COPD
continued

6. Sitting to standing:

Using a dining chair, sit, stand, sit, allowing ten seconds from start to completion. Repeat continuously for 40 seconds for a total of five repetitions. Repeat three times with a short rest period after each procedure.

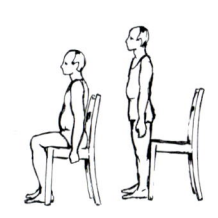

7. Quadriceps exercise:

Sitting on chair straighten right knee, tense thigh muscles, hold for count of four, then relax gradually over a further four seconds to a total of five repetitions over 40 seconds. Repeat the exercise three times with short rest periods in between sets. Repeat with left leg.

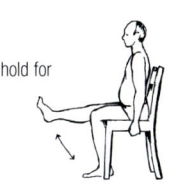

8. Calf exercises:

Holding onto back of chair, go up on toes, return to floor taking eight to ten seconds to complete procedure. Repeat continuously for 40 seconds.

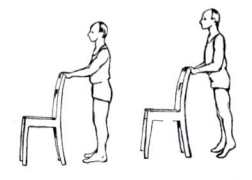

9. Walking on the spot:

Holding onto the back of a chair, allow one knee to bend, keeping toes on the floor. Bend other knee, while straightening first knee. Allow four seconds for complete procedure. Repeat this bending/straightening of knees (i.e. walking on the spot) keeping toes on the floor continuously for 40 seconds to a total of ten repetitions. Repeat the exercise three times with short rest periods after each procedure.

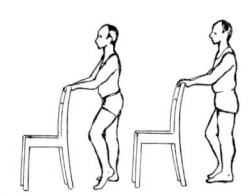

10. Step ups:

Step up with the right foot onto step; then bring up left foot. Step down with right foot and then with left foot. Allow four seconds for the complete procedure and repeat continuously for 40 seconds. Repeat the exercise three times with short rest periods in between sets.

NOTES
- Encourage patients to keep as active as possible and exercise to the limits of their ability
- Walking is an excellent exercise for COPD patients

Breathing exercises

Need for breathing exercises

- Breathless patients hold the upper chest and shoulder girdle in a position of inspiration and overwork the accessory muscles of inspiration, thus requiring greater energy
- Taking deep breaths can increase the work of breathing and worsen the sensation of breathlessness
- Breathing exercises can give back an element of control over breathing and give patients confidence in their ability to exercise more.

Teaching breathing control

- The aim is to minimize the work of breathing and encourage a return to a normal pattern of respiration
- Reducing the effort of breathing is achieved by gentle breathing
- This is a passive exercise, involving relaxing the upper chest and shoulders
- Patients may maximize effective breathing control by assuming a position of relaxation.

Positions of relaxation

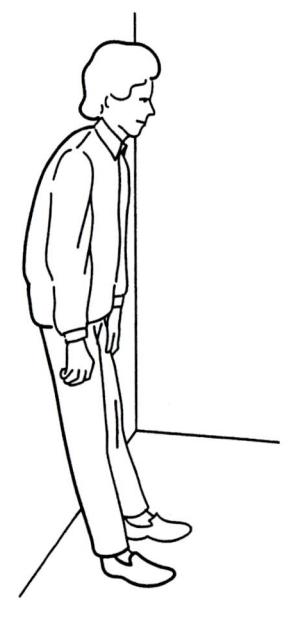

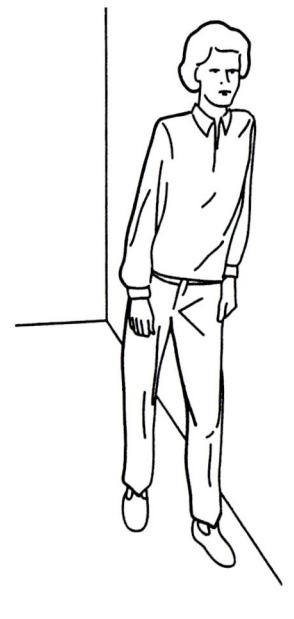

Forward lean standing position against wall

Sideways forward lean standing position against a wall

Breathing exercises continued

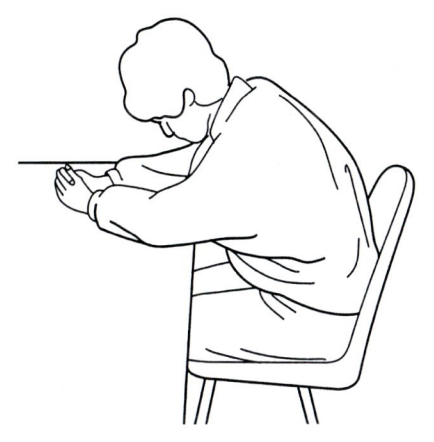

Forward lean sitting position

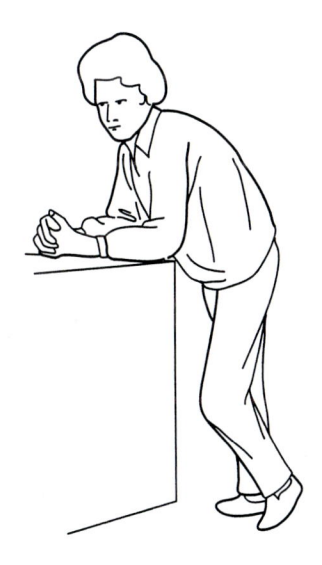

Forward lean standing position

- Emphasize breathing rhythms:
  - While walking, breathe in for one step, out for two
  - While sitting or standing breathe in for two seconds, out for three seconds
- Gentle pursed lip breathing may help with breathing control; forceful exhalation increases airway collapse and air trapping.

Breathing exercises continued

Respiratory muscle training
- Specific exercises for strengthening respiratory muscles may be part of a formal pulmonary rehabilitation programme.

Nutrition

It has been estimated that around 21% of individuals with COPD in the UK are at risk of malnutrition. The causes of malnutrition in COPD patients are varied and the consequences are significant. Malnutrition may develop gradually over several years or might develop or progress following exacerbations. Screening should take place on first contact with a patient and/or upon clinical concern e.g. recent exacerbation, change in social or psychological status. A review should take place at least annually and more frequently if risk of malnutrition is identified. For further information on identifying and managing disease related malnutrition, please see 'Managing Adult Malnutrition in the Community' (www.malnutritionpathway.co.uk).

- Underweight patients should be advised to maximize their calorie intake by eating small, frequent meals and resting before and after eating. Nutritional supplements may be helpful
- Overweight or obese patients should be given dietary advice, but fear of further weight gain should not be a reason for avoiding smoking cessation.

Self–management plans
- Good self-management can reduce complications, promote symptom control and improve quality of life
- The main aim is to prevent exacerbations and allow patients to develop the skills to recognise and treat an exacerbation at an early stage
- Patients who experience frequent exacerbations may benefit from having a course of antibiotics and/or oral corticosteroids at home as part of a self-management plan
- Patients should be taught how to respond promptly to the symptoms of an exacerbation by:
  - Adjusting their bronchodilators to control their symptoms
  - Starting antibiotics if their sputum becomes purulent
  - Starting oral corticosteroids if their increased breathlessness interferes with their normal activities of daily living and does not respond to increased bronchodilator therapy
- Patients need clear instructions on when they should call their doctor or nurse

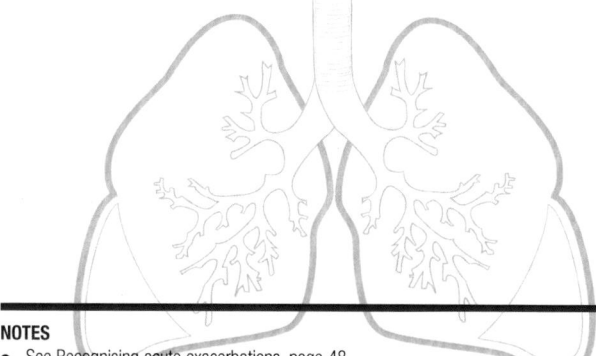

NOTES
- See Recognising acute exacerbations, page 48
- Respiratory mucus clearing devices such as the Flutter or Acapella may also be helpful

Managing stable COPD

Aims of management

- Best control of symptoms
- Prevention of deterioration
- Prevention of complications
- Improved quality of life for patients and their families.

Setting objectives and monitoring response follow–up
Page 34

Maximizing the effectiveness of pharmacotherapy
Page 35

Medications
Pages 36-41

Medication Delivery
Page 42

Oxygen therapy
Pages 43-44

Surgery
Page 45

Routine follow-up
Page 46

Self-management – particularly smoking cessation – is at least as important as the medical management of COPD – see pages 22-25.

Setting objectives and monitoring response to treatment

- Monitoring the impact of treatment on patient/family life is more important than monitoring lung function
- Changes in the sense of wellbeing, exercise capacity and freedom from exacerbations may be apparent without measurable changes in lung function.

Setting objectives
- Understand the patient's goals, expectations and motivations
- Overall aim is to keep the patient functioning within the home setting for as long as possible
- Early diagnosis, with help to quit smoking, may prevent progression of mild COPD
- Offer education on causes and progression of COPD
- Agree a management plan
- Set and monitor realistic goals, including smoking cessation.

Monitoring response to treatment
- Document effects of each change in management in terms of disability (see pages 17-18 for measurements of disability and page 35 for questions to ask)
- Assess for signs of depression and isolation and encourage patient to accept appropriate interventions
- Arrange home visits for patients with severe COPD to help with psychosocial problems as well as respiratory care.

Taking action, educating people and transforming lives worldwide

NOTES
- For spirometry, see page 6
- For assessment of quality of life and breathlessness, see pages 16-18
- For improving self-management, see pages 28-32

Maximising the effectiveness of pharmacotherapy

NICE 2019 recommends that before pharmacotherapy is considered, attention should be paid to supporting people to quit smoking, reminding them to have a flu jab and a pneumonia jab and encouraging them to attend pulmonary rehabilitation, where appropriate.

Objectives of pharmacotherapy

- To maximise symptom control and reduce exacerbations by choosing the best medications for each patient
- To limit the medications taken by each patient to those which have demonstrated a positive effect.

Bronchodilators

- It is thought that bronchodilators work by reducing overinflation and permitting better respiratory muscle function
- Increasing the dose of bronchodilators may be symptomatically helpful for some patients but has to be balanced against the risk of side effects. It may be better to consider another class of bronchodilator
- Individual COPD patients may have a better response to different classes of bronchodilators such as long-acting beta-agonists or long-acting anti-muscarinics. Assessment of effect should be measured in changes in symptoms and measuring improvement in quality of life.

Assess response by asking:

'Has your treatment made a difference to you?'
'Is your breathing easier in any way?'
'Can you do some things now that you couldn't do before, or the same things but faster?'
'Can you do the same things as before but are now less breathless when you do them?'
'Has your sleep improved?'

Response can also be assessed by asking patients to grade effectiveness on a four-point scale as:

Ineffective
Satisfactory
Effective
Very effective

Response can also be assessed by recalculating the CAT score using COPD assessment tool.

Managing stable COPD

Medications

Bronchodilator therapy

- Bronchodilators are the cornerstone of symptoms therapy for COPD
- They are effective at reducing symptoms even though they may not significantly improve the spirometry readings
- Correct medication, dose and timing must be tailored to the individual.

NICE (2019) recommends that bronchodilators should be the mainstay of COPD care and that inhaled corticosteroids are primarily indicated for people with a reversible element to their condition. If a short–acting bronchodilator is not enough to control symptoms, NICE recommends moving straight to a dual bronchodilator. GOLD takes a more tailored approach. There are pros and cons to both of these approaches.

Short-acting, inhaled beta$_2$ agonists (SABAs)

- Available in metered dose inhaler (MDI), a wide variety of dry powder inhalers, breath–actuated inhalers and solutions for nebulisers
- Use as required for symptom relief or regularly
- Initially use 2 inhalations (200 mcg) salbutamol up to 4 times daily, or terbutaline (500mcg) up to four times day
- Side effects of tremor and palpitation may develop; care required with high doses in elderly patients with known cardiac history. (Measure potassium levels twice yearly in patients on high–dose beta$_2$ agonists: hypokalaemia may be a problem, particularly if the patient is also on a diuretic such as furosemide).

Long-acting inhaled beta$_2$ agonists (LABAs)

- Formoterol, salmeterol, olodaterol and indacaterol are licensed for use in COPD
- They improve exercise tolerance, symptoms and health–related quality of life and reduce exacerbation rates
- Long-acting bronchodilator(s) should be used when short-acting agents fail to control symptoms adequately
- The onset of action differs between the LABAs.

Short-acting muscarinic antagonists (SAMAs)

- Ipratropium bromide (Atrovent) is available as an MDI, and solution for nebulisation
- Muscarinic antagonists may be as, or more effective than beta$_2$ agonists in some patients with COPD
- Use 2-4 inhalations of ipratropium bromide 3-4 times daily but NICE suggests using a long-acting muscarinic antagonist as an alternative.

Long-acting muscarinic antagonists (LAMAs)

Long-acting muscarinic antagonists (LAMAs) include tiotropium, aclidinium, glycopyrronium and umeclidinium. Aclidinium is taken twice daily, the others are all once daily treatments. They are available in a range of devices to suit different patients. LAMAs may improve symptoms of breathlessness and quality of life scores. Some have been shown to reduce exacerbation risk.

Dual bronchodilators

Dual bronchodilators are made up of a long-acting beta2 agonist with a long-acting muscarinic antagonist. Using these two therapies together in one inhaler may help to improve quality of life and symptoms of breathlessness. Dual bronchodilators include vilanterol/umeclidinium (Anoro) in the Ellipta device; formoterol/aclidinium (Duaklir) in the Genuair device, glycopyrronium/indacaterol (Ultibro), in the Breezhaler device, and tiotropium/olodaterol (Spiolto) in the Respimat device.

Oral theophylline

- This has a narrow therapeutic index so best reserved for patients whose symptoms are inadequately controlled with other treatments
- Cardiac side effects and drug interactions can be troublesome, particularly in the elderly
- Monitoring is required: blood levels should be between 10-20mg/L
- Theophylline blood levels are decreased by smoking, increased by smoking cessation and by influenza vaccination. Other significant interactions may occur with a variety of medicines
- Always check for interactions in the *British National Formulary*
- Oral theophyllines should be prescribed by brand to optimise stability of blood levels

NOTES
- Theophylline interactions are listed in the *British National Formulary*

Bronchodilator therapy continued

GOLD–towards personalised care

GOLD (2019) guidelines recognise differences in patients with COPD and describe the different phenotypes on the basis of symptoms and frequency of exacerbations. This is a move away from using lung function as a guide to severity and treatment on the basis that there is poor correlation between lung function and symptoms. The GOLD ABCD algorithm allows different presentations of COPD to be categorised and treated appropriately.

Categorise according to mMRC or CAT score and frequency of exacerbations:

- Assess symptom severity using modified MRC or CAT scores (along the bottom of the grid)
- Then add exacerbation history (on the right hand side of the grid) based on whether they have had 0-1 exacerbations, one severe exacerbation requiring hospitalisation or two or more exacerbations of any severity
- Patients will end up in category A, B, C or D.

GOLD 2019

	mMRC 0-1 CAT < 10	mMRC ≥ 2 CAT ≥ 10	RISK Exacerbation History
	C	D	≥2 or 1 requiring admission to hospital
	A	B	1 0

SYMPTOMS
mMRC or CAT score

GOLD GROUP	INITIAL THERAPY	OTHER OPTIONS
A	SABA, SAMA	LAMA or LABA
B	LAMA or LABA	LAMA + LABA
C	LAMA	LAMA + LABA ICS/LABA
D	LAMA + LABA	ICS/LABA +/- LAMA

Inhaled corticosteroids (ICS)

- ICS are only licensed to be used in combination with long-acting bronchodilators so ICS are not licensed in COPD as monotherapy
- ICS do not significantly reduce the rate of lung function decline in COPD at any stage of the disease
- GOLD (2019) suggests that eosinophil levels can identify those who might benefit most from an ICS/LABA. The GOLD guidelines state that if eosinophil levels are:
- <100 eosinophils per µL – no role for ICS
- >100 plus history of acute exacerbations of COPD (two or more in 12 months) there is evidence for ICS
- >300 – evidence for ICS, even if no history of acute exacerbations
- ICS may not be licensed in patients with moderate airflow obstruction (FEV_1 greater than 50% predicted)
- ICS may reduce exacerbation rates and the decline in health status associated with frequent exacerbations
- Patients with clear features of asthma, or who have developed fixed airflow obstruction as a result of long-standing asthma should be treated with ICS in line with conventional asthma guidelines.

Combination inhaled steroids and long-acting beta$_2$ agonists

- Combination inhalers: licensed combinations for use in COPD include:
  budesonide/formoterol 400/12mcg (Symbicort 400 Turbohaler) 1 puff bd
  budesonide/formoterol 200/6mcg (Symbicort 200 Turbohaler) 2 puffs bd
  budesonide/formoterol 200/6mcg (Symbicort 200 pMDI) 2 puffs bd
  budesonide/formoterol fumarate 320/9mcg (DuoResp Spiromax) 1 puff bd
  budesonide/formoterol 160/4.5mcg (DuoResp Spiromax) 2 puffs bd
  budesonide/formoterol 320/9mcg Fobumix Easyhaler one puff bd
  fluticasone proprionate/salmeterol 500/50mcg (Seretide 500 Accuhaler) 1 puff bd
  fluticasone proprionate/salmeterol 500/50mcg (Aerivio Spiromax) 1 puff bd
  fluticasone proprionate/salmeterol 500/50mcg (Airflusal Forspiro) 1 puff bd
  fluticasone furoate/vilanterol 92/22mcg (Relvar Ellipta) 1 puff once daily
  beclometasone/formoterol 100/6mcg (Fostair pMDI) 2 puffs bd
  beclometasone/formoterol 100/6mcg (Fostair NEXThaler) 2 puffs bd
- Studies have shown that these combinations are effective at improving symptoms and reducing the frequency of exacerbations
- High dose ICS should not be necessary for most patients
- Patients over 65 on high dose inhaled steroids or oral steroids should routinely receive osteoporosis prophylaxis. All patients on high dose inhaled steroids should be warned of the potential side effects of this treatment, particularly osteoporosis, type 2 diabetes and non–fatal pneumonia.

Triple therapy in one device

The GOLD guidelines suggest that some patients who have category D COPD will benefit from triple therapy: an ICS, LABA and LAMA. In 2017, two triple therapy inhalers were launched. Trimbow™ contains extra fine beclometasone with formoterol and glycopyrronium (i.e. Fostair with an additional LAMA) in a metered dose inhaler. The drug is licensed to use as maintenance therapy in people with moderate to severe COPD who are not adequately treated with an ICS/LABA combination and is taken as a set dose of 2 puffs twice daily. Trelegy™ contains fluticasone furoate, vilanterol and umeclidinium in the Ellipta device and is taken as a set dose of 1 puff once a day.

Oral corticosteroids (OCS)

- There is no evidence that long-term oral corticosteroids have any benefit in COPD. They should be avoided due to significant side effects.

Mucolytics

- Mucolytic agents reduce the viscosity of mucus in the airways
- A trial of mucolytics can be considered for patients with chronic productive cough
- Therapy should be continued if the patient reports an improvement in their symptoms.

PDE 4 inhibitors

- This drug class is not used very often in the UK due to side effects although it is mentioned in the GOLD guidelines and may be initiated in secondary care.

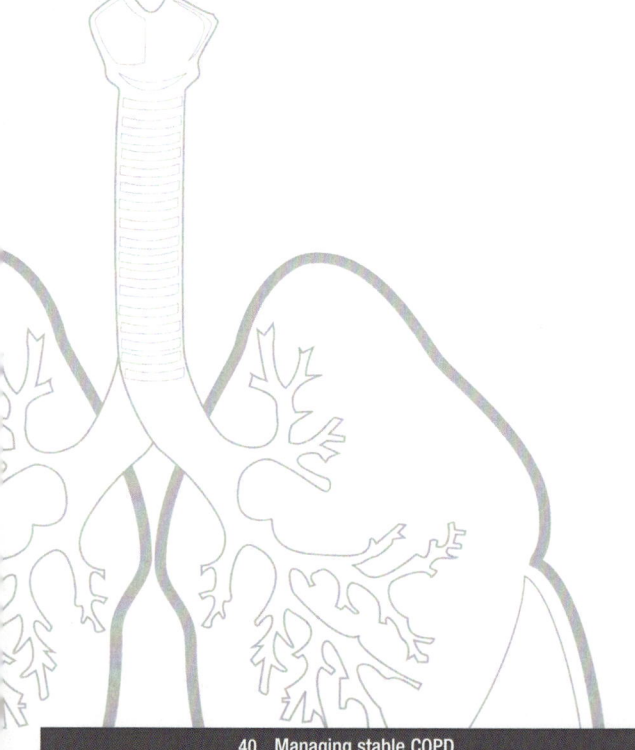

Other medications

Other anti-inflammatories
- Leukotriene receptor antagonists do not have any beneficial effect for patients with COPD.

Antibiotics
- Antibiotics may be used in acute infective exacerbations of COPD. Sputum colour and CRP levels may help to identify those people who are most likely to benefit from antibiotic therapy. Local guidelines should be used to inform treatment choices.

Anti-depressants
- Depression is very common, particularly in advanced COPD
- Depression should be assessed by quality of life or depression questionnaires
- Standard anti-depressant medication is safe for use in COPD and can be very effective in improving quality of life
- Some patients may benefit from talking therapies, cognitive behavioural therapy or social prescribing interventions.

Vaccinations and anti-viral therapy
- Annual influenza vaccination can reduce serious illness and death in COPD patients
- Annual influenza vaccination is recommended by NICE and the Department of Health and Social Care
- There is less evidence for the efficacy of pneumococcal vaccination in COPD patients, but vaccination is safe and is recommended by NICE and Department of Health and Social Care
- The anti-influenza treatments, zanamavir or oseltamavir, are recommended by NICE for COPD patients with influenza-like illness if they are able to start treatment within 48 hours of the onset of symptoms. However, there is limited evidence for their use.

Other health maintenance issues
- Adequate calcium and vitamin D are important, particularly in patients on high dose ICS or oral corticosteroids
- Monitoring for osteoporosis and osteoporosis prophylaxis may need to be considered for patients who require frequent short courses of oral steroids, or who are taking high dose inhaled repeated courses of oral corticosteroids.

Tools such as these FRAX: https://www.sheffield.ac.uk/FRAX/tool.aspx or QFracture: http://www.qfracture.org/ may be useful in identifying people at risk of osteoporotic fractures.

NOTES
- For determining the effectiveness of various medications, see page 35
- For assessing breathlessness and quality of life, see pages 16-18

Medication delivery

Inhalation devices include:
- Metered dose inhalers (pMDIs) preferably with a spacer
- Breath–actuated devices
- Dry powder inhalers (DPIs)
- Soft mist inhalers
- Nebulisers

The main errors in delivery device use relate to problems with inspiratory flow, inhalation duration and coordination.

- Consideration should be given to the patient's ability, preference and lifestyle when selecting a device
- Inhaler technique should be checked at each visit
- Technique and adherence should be assessed before concluding current therapy is insufficient.

Inhalation technique
Generation of a drug preparation for inhalation requires energy. The source of the energy varies depending on the device used:
- In a pMDI the aerosol is generated by the evaporation of the propellant
- In a dry powder inhaler (DPI) the energy is generated by the inspiratory effort of the patient and comes from the flow of air through the device that the patient produces
- In a nebuliser the energy is provided by the driving gas (jet nebuliser), or from the ultrasonic vibration of a Piezo crystal (ultrasonic and mesh nebuliser).

All inhaler devices require different amounts of effort and individual patient variables will determine whether inhaler technique is effective or not.

Long–term nebulised bronchodilators
- Nebulisers may be required for administration of high–dose bronchodilator therapy in patients with distressing and disabling breathlessness despite maximum therapy with hand–held inhalers
- Long–term nebulised therapy should not be given without assessment by a specialist. Assessment should confirm that nebulised therapy produces one of the following
  - Reduction in symptoms
  - Increase in ability to perform activities of daily living
  - Increased exercise capacity
  - Improved lung function
- The ability of the patient and their carers to use and care for the equipment needs to be assessed
- The patient should be provided with all necessary equipment and disposables (replacement tubing, nebuliser sets, mouthpieces/masks and filters) as well as supportive services: servicing, advice, education and support.

Oxygen therapy

Long-term oxygen therapy (LTOT)

- Long-term administration of oxygen has been shown to prolong life in patients with COPD and chronic hypoxia
- Patients must be assessed for LTOT by a specialist
- Patients with an FEV_1 of 30-49% predicted should be referred for assessment if they have one or more of:
  - cyanosis
  - polycythaemia
  - raised jugular venous pressure (JVP)
  - oxygen saturation measured with a pulse oximeter (SaO_2) 92% or less when stable and breathing air
- All patients with severe COPD and/or very severe airflow obstruction ($FEV_1 < 30\%$ predicted) should be considered for LTOT
- The benefit of oxygen is seen with daily use for 15 hours or more
- Assessment for LTOT should be made when the patient is clinically stable and at least four weeks after an exacerbation
- Continued smoking is not an absolute contraindication for LTOT, but patients who continue to smoke must be warned about the risks of fire and explosion
- There is evidence of reduced benefit from LTOT in smokers.

Criteria for LTOT

- Patients should be taking optimum drug therapy
  - PaO_2 less than 7.3kPa when breathing air

OR

  - PaO_2 7.3-8kPa and one of:
  - Polycythaemia
  - Nocturnal hypoxia
  - Pulmonary hypertension
- Arterial blood gases must be assessed on at least 2 occasions at least three weeks apart.

Assessing patients on LTOT

- Once on LTOT, patients should be reviewed at least annually by a practitioner familiar with LTOT
- Annual review must include measurement of SaO_2 with a pulse oximeter

Delivery systems for LTOT

- Oxygen must be given for a minimum of 15 hours a day
- Nasal cannulae (nasal prongs) are generally used as they allow the patient to eat with oxygen in situ and are less intrusive

Ambulatory oxygen therapy

- COPD patients receiving LTOT who wish to continue with oxygen outside the home may benefit from a portable oxygen supply
- Patients who meet the following criteria may be suitable:
  - Severe breathlessness
  - Oxygen desaturation, and
  - Improved exercise capacity when ambulatory oxygen is provided

Oxygen therapy continued

Short-burst oxygen therapy

Short-burst oxygen is one of the most expensive therapies for COPD. There is a lack of evidence for its effectiveness. Some of its apparent benefits may be due to the simple cooling effects of the stream of gas on the face. Some studies have shown that an electric fan blowing onto the face can be just as effective in this respect.
Short–burst oxygen should therefore only be used in palliative care.

Non-invasive ventilation (NIV)

- NIV is a method of providing ventilatory support without the need to sedate and intubate the patient. It is generally delivered from a tight-fitting nasal or facial mask.

  COPD patients with chronic hypercapnia may benefit from ventilatory support.

  The NICE guidelines recommend:
- Optimally treated patients with chronic hypercapnic respiratory failure, who have required ventilation during an exacerbation, or who are hypercapnic or acidotic on LTOT, should be referred to a specialist centre for assessment for long-term NIV.

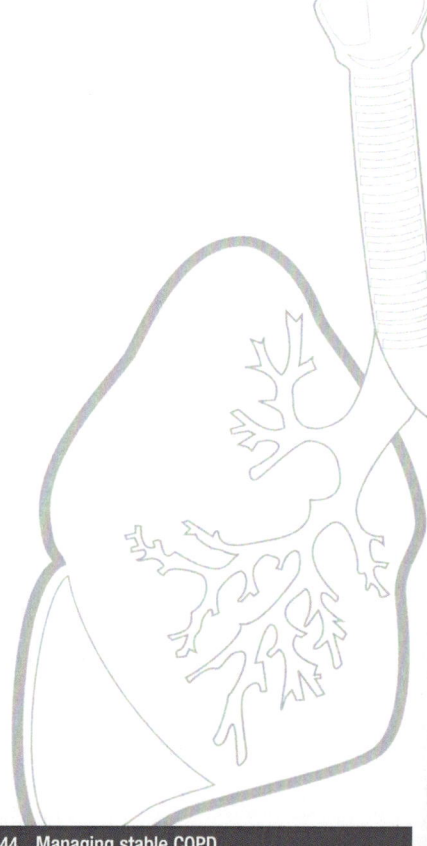

Surgery

Surgery may be an option for a few, carefully selected COPD patients.
It is most frequently offered to those with disabling COPD and no co-morbid conditions.

Lung volume reduction (LVR) surgery

The worst affected area of the lung is excised, allowing re-expansion of the less badly affected areas. This has the effect of improving respiratory mechanics and reducing breathlessness.

Bullectomy

Bullae are large, cyst-like, emphysematous spaces in the lung. They can lead to compression of relatively normal lung tissue. Excision of a bulla can reduce breathlessness and improve lung function in some patients.

Lung transplant

Patients over the age of 50 years are not usually considered for lung transplantation, so this option is most appropriate for alpha 1 antitrypsin deficient patients as they tend to present with severe COPD at a young age. The main technique is single lung transplant although double lung transplant is occasionally performed. UK survival figures are 60% at three years.

Other options

Other surgical options are being trialled, including lung volume reduction coils which reduce hyperinflation. This procedure is done via bronchoscopy and appears to offer significant benefits to patients with emphysema.

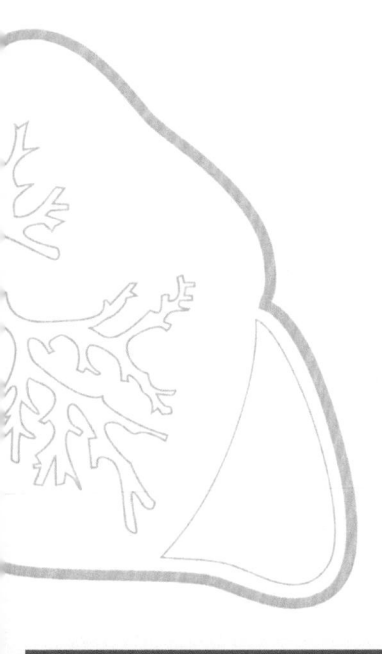

Routine follow-up

MILD/MODERATE COPD	SEVERE/VERY SEVERE COPD

FREQUENCY

6-12 MONTHS	3-6 MONTHS

CLINICAL ASSESSMENT

Smoking status and desire to stop	**Smoking status and desire to stop**
Symptom control Breathlessness Exercise tolerance Exacerbation frequency	**Symptom control** Breathlessness Exercise tolerance Exacerbation frequency
Please consider Effects of drug therapy Inhaler technique Need for specialist referral Need for pulmonary rehabilitation Inhaler technique	**Please consider** Cor pulmonale and need for LTOT Nutritional status Presence of depression Effects of drug therapy Inhaler technique Need for specialist referral Social services Occupational therapy Need for pulmonary rehabilitation

Managing the acute exacerbation

Recognising acute exacerbations
Page 48

Treatment in the community
Page 49

Treatment in the hospital
Page 50

Hospital–at–home and assisted discharge schemes
Page 51

Recognising acute exacerbations

- Acute exacerbations present as a worsening of symptoms, beyond normal day–to–day variation
- The change in symptoms often necessitates a change in medication
- The new event may be due to viral or bacterial infection or related to poor air quality
- Exacerbations are distressing and disruptive for patients
- They are significant events that result in worsening prognosis.

Important signs and symptoms include:

- Worsening breathlessness
- Increase in sputum purulence
- Increase in sputum volume

They may also be associated with

- Increased cough
- Upper airway symptoms (e.g. colds, sore throat)
- Increased wheeze
- Chest tightness
- Reduced exercise tolerance
- Increased fatigue

Exacerbations may precipitate cor pulmonale and respiratory failure leading to

- Fluid retention
- Cyanosis and SaO_2 <90%
- Acute confusion

Pulse oximeters should be available in both hospital and community settings. Although they give no information about CO_2 levels or acidosis (pH) they are an important part of assessing an exacerbation of COPD.

Assessment of severity of exacerbation

Some exacerbations are mild and self–limiting. Others are severe and carry a risk of death. They may necessitate hospitalisation.

The presence of any of the following indicates a severe exacerbation:

- Marked breathlessness
- Increased respiratory rate
- Pursed lip breathing
- Use of accessory muscles at rest
- Acute confusion
- New onset cyanosis
- New onset peripheral oedema
- Marked reduction in activities of daily living

Differential diagnoses to consider

- Pneumonia
- Pneumothorax
- Left ventricular failure/pulmonary oedema
- Pulmonary embolus
- Lung cancer
- Upper airway obstruction
- Pleural effusion

Treatment in the community

Bronchodilators

The use of bronchodilators should be optimised. Those currently prescribed should be used at high doses and others may need to be added.

- Nebulised bronchodilators may need to be considered if high doses are required and the patient is unable to use a hand-held device.

Corticosteroids

- A short course of oral corticosteroids should be given if breathlessness significantly interferes with a patient's normal daily activities
- NICE suggest prednisolone 30mg daily for 7-14 days. However, evidence suggests that prolonged courses do not give increased benefit and recent evidence from the REDUCE study suggests 40mg given for five days may offer the greatest benefit with the lowest risk
- There is no need to taper the dose if the course does not exceed 14 days

Antibiotic therapy

- Antibiotics should be used if the exacerbation is associated with sputum purulence
- Antibiotics should also be used if there are clinical signs of pneumonia or consolidation increased on the chest X-ray, even if the sputum is not purulent
- Initial therapy should follow guidance from local microbiologists
  – usually an aminopenicillin, a macrolide or tetracycline.

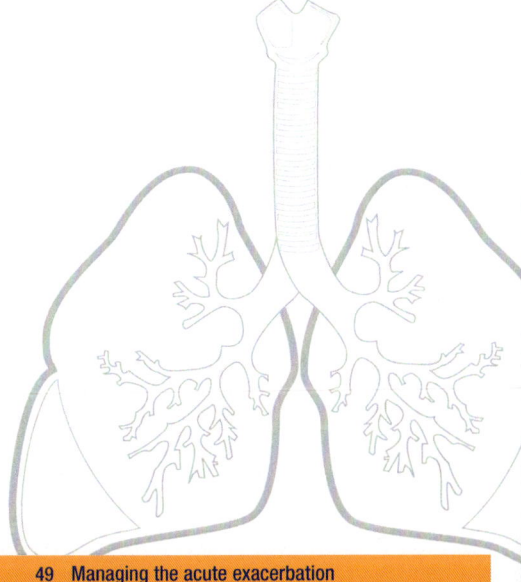

Treatment in the hospital

Factors to consider when deciding whether to treat an exacerbation at home or to admit the patient to hospital:

Indicator	Treat at home	Treat at hospital
Able to cope at home	Yes	No
Breathlessness	Mild	Severe
General condition	Good	Poor/deteriorating
Level of activity	Normal	Poor/bed bound
Cyanosis	No	Yes
Worsening peripheral oedema	No	Yes
Level of consciousness	Normal	Impaired
Already on LTOT	No	Yes
Social circumstances	Good	Living alone/not coping
Acute confusion	No	Yes
Rapid rate of onset	No	Yes
Significant co-morbidities (particularly cardiac or insulin-dependent diabetes)	No	Yes
Changes on chest x-ray	No	Yes
Arterial pH level	≥ 7.35	<7.35
Arterial PaO_2	≥ 7 kPa	< 7 kPa

All patients referred to hospital should have:
- Chest X-ray
- Arterial blood gases measured and inspired O_2 concentration recorded
- An ECG – to exclude co-morbidities
- A full blood count and urea and electrolytes
- A sputum sample sent for analysis if sputum is purulent

Drug therapy in hospital
- Oral corticosteroids should be given to all patients admitted to hospital with an exacerbation of COPD
- The same principles apply to bronchodilator therapy in the community and the hospital
- Serum potassium may need to be monitored in patients on high doses of nebulised beta$_2$ agonist bronchodilators
- Antibiotic therapy will need to be reviewed according to the result of sputum microscopy and culture.

Oxygen therapy

The aim of oxygen therapy is to maintain adequate oxygenation without precipitating respiratory acidosis or hypercapnia in acute exacerbations.

- SaO_2 should be monitored
- A target saturation range of 88-92% in the acutely ill COPD patient should be aimed for until arterial blood gases are undertaken. Following blood gases with no history of hypercapnia and normal $PaCO_2$, the target saturation range should be 94-98%
- Oxygen should be given at approximately 40% and titrated up if the SaO_2 falls below 90%, and titrated down if the patient becomes drowsy or SaO_2 exceeds 93-4%
- Blood gases should be monitored regularly according to response to treatment.

If the patient is hypercapnic $PaCO_2$ > 6Kpa and acidotic pH <7.35 consider NIV especially if acidosis has persisted for more than 30 minutes despite appropriate treatment.

Non–invasive ventilation (NIV)

- NIV is the treatment of choice for persistent hypercapnic respiratory failure during exacerbations that have not responded to optimal medical therapy
- Before NIV is commenced a clear plan covering what to do in the event of treatment failure should be agreed.

Invasive ventilation may be needed for some patients if they are unable to tolerate NIV. For others, NIV will be the 'ceiling' of therapy.

Hospital-at-home and assisted discharge schemes

Hospital-at-home and assisted discharge schemes are safe and effective. They are an alternative way of caring for patients with uncomplicated exacerbations of COPD who would otherwise need to be admitted.

Patient preferences about treatment at home or in hospital will need to be considered, but such schemes are generally well received.

Education for Health training programme

Education for Health provides a wide range of education and training across cardiovascular, diabetes, respiratory and professional skills, including half–day and one-day workshops, Diploma, Degree and Masters level modules and programmes.

Workshops

Our workshops combine group work and practical demonstrations, covering the fundamentals of diagnosis, management and treatment. Our modules are designed for both primary and secondary health care professionals working with patients with long-term conditions.

The following workshops are currently available: ACD of Hypertension
- Allergy and Anaphylaxis • Aspire to Inspire • Assessing and Managing Joint Pain Problems in Primary Care: the knee • Asthma Update • Atrial Fibrillation • Breaking Bad News • CBT: An introduction to the principles of Cognitive Behavioural Therapy
- Communication for Non-Malignant Palliative Care: Masterclass for GPs • COPD Update
- Core Consultation Skills • Dementia • Essentials of Allergic Rhinitis and its Impact on Asthma • Essentials of Asthma • Essentials of COPD • Essentials of Primary Care Nursing • Homecare and the COPD Patient • Hypertension in Practice
- Introduction to Diabetes • Introduction to Heart Failure • Introduction to Self–Management and Behaviour Change • Non–Malignant Palliative Care
- Paediatric Asthma • Putting Prevention First • Reading and Understanding Research Papers • Smoking Cessation • Spirometry for HCAs • Spirometry
- Stroke • Tackling CVD Risk • Weight Management

Diploma and Degree programmes

All Diploma, Degree and Masters level modules are delivered by eLearning, with many of the modules also including study days across the UK. These modules can be undertaken as stand-alone modules or students can join our programmes to work towards a DipHE, BSc or MSc qualification. The Diploma and Degree modules (Levels 5 and 6) are validated by The Open University and the Masters (Level 7) modules are accredited by the University of Hertfordshire. We also have a small number of quality-assured professional development modules without academic credits.

The following workshops are currently available:

Degree Modules

- Allergy • Asthma • Atrial Fibrillation • Bringing Evidence to Practice
- Cardiovascular Disease Risk • COPD • Coronary Heart Disease • Diabetes
- Heart Failure • Holistic Care for People Living with Long–Term Conditions • Hypertension
- Smoking Cessation • Spirometry • Stroke in Primary Care • Tuberculosis

Masters Level Modules

These are accredited by the University of Hertfordshire and include modules relating to asthma, COPD, respiratory ethics, respiratory assessment and examination and others.

Education for Health courses are run at our venues across England and Scotland. We can also bring training to your local area anywhere in the UK if you have 15+ people interested.

Further information is available on the Education for Health website:
www.educationforhealth.org

Contact:
Email: info@educationforhealth.org   Telephone: +44 (0) 1926 493313

Useful address

British Lung Foundation (BLF)
Information on COPD www.blf.org.uk

Other 'Simply' pocket books

The 'Simply' series of practical pocket books offer bite–size evidence-based guidance on the practical issues facing healthcare professionals when caring for patients in everyday practice.

To view the full range of titles in our 'Simply' book series, or to place an order please visit www.educationforhealth.org or ring 01926 493313.

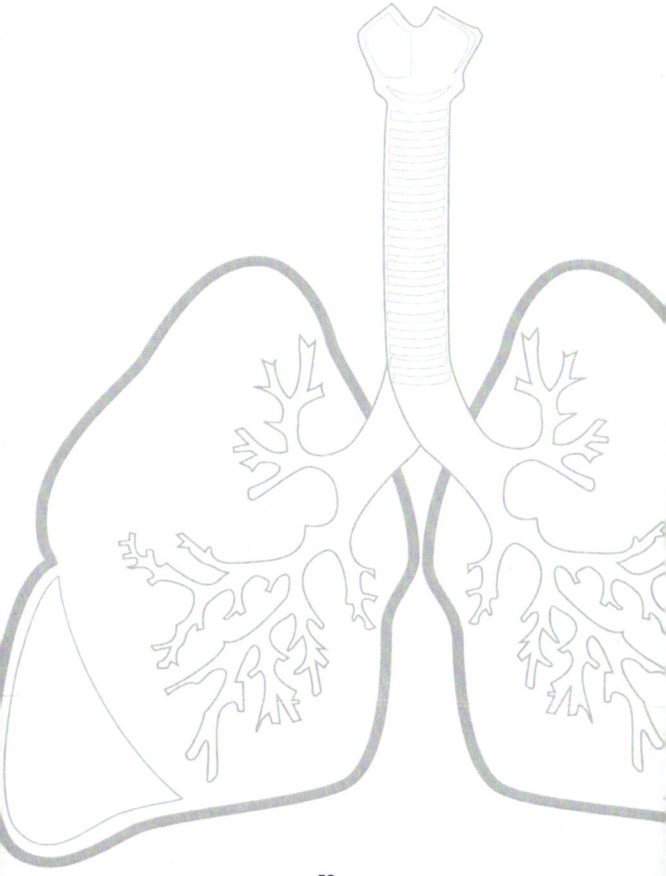

Taking **action**, educating people and transforming lives worldwide